BED-WETTING ENURESIS

by

Dr. Farokh J. Master

L.C.E.H. (Bom.), Gold Medalist ;
Honarary Homoeopathic Consultant, Bombay Hospital & Medical Research Centre ;
Lecturer in Medicine, C.M. P.H. Medical College, Bombay.

Foreword by :

Dr. Jugal Kishore,

B. Sc., D.M.S., M.D. (Hon.)

B. JAIN PUBLISHERS (P) Ltd.

USA — EUROPE — INDIA

8th Impression: 2012

Note From the Publishers
Any information given in this book is not intended to be taken as a replacement for medical advice. Any person with a condition requiring medical attention should consult a qualified practitioner or therapist.

Published by Kuldeep Jain for
B. JAIN PUBLISHERS (P) LTD.
1921/10, Chuna Mandi, Paharganj, New Delhi 110 055 (INDIA)
Tel.: +91-11-4567 1000 Fax: +91-11-4567 1010
Email: info@bjain.com Website: **www.bjain.com**

Printed in India by
J.J. Offset Printers

ISBN 978-81-319-0016-1

FOREWORD

It is a pleasure writing a foreword of this booklet written by Dr. Farokh Master who has taken lot of pains for collecting material on the subject. Since Enuresis Nocturia is a problem so commonly met with in every day experience of every physician, it is welcome to have an informative booklet on this subject.

Apart from giving the history and causes of this problem, he has compiled the repertorial analysis of various remedies indicated for this condition. He could have avoided one or two isolated rubrics for certain conditions, *e.g.*, under 56. Enuresis of Children—Benz. acid and Kali-phos. are given and under 55. Enuresis, wetting of bed—Hep. s. is given. He has, however, given classified indications for commonly indicated remedies. I am sure the book will be warmly received by the profession.

New Delhi
The 10th April, 1985

Dr. Jugal Kishore
B. Sc., D.M.S., M.D. (Hom.),
President, Central Council of Homoeopathy ;
Past-President, Hom. Med. Asso. of India ;
Hony. Hom. Physician to the President of India.

Dated [illegible] April 1983

[illegible]

Past President, Homoeopathic Medical Assn. of India

PREFACE

The childhood shows the man, as morning shows the day.

Milton : *Paradise Regained*

In preparing the manuscript of this work, I have followed the lines laid out by the American College of Psychiatry for the treatment of enuresis.

I was tempted to write this book after I saw in my practice that out of every ten children who came to my clinic atleast two of them were suffering from bed-wetting.

This problem till to date was very poorly understood by me therefore I decided to read (books referred are mentioned in Bibliography) and then to save time of the busy practitioner I have put the matter in a condensed form. For easy reference of remedy I have described the remedy in tabulated form, aided by a small repertory.

I have been aided in seeing this edition through the press by the efficient help of Dr. (Miss) Archana C. Maniar and Dr. Nimesh P. Sukhla. They have lightened the labour of making the manuscript more acceptable to the profession and I desire to express my hearty appreciation of this kind and helpful service.

Bed-wetting being one of the commonest problems as I found in my clinics (2 out of every 10 children had come across in my practice), I was forced to take up a detailed study and interest in this subject as not only this complaint formed an embarrassing situation for the tiny tots but I found it to bear a deep traumatic psychological influence on these subjects especially when the younger one was in a position to acheive a control over his or her bladder earlier than the older one.

This problem till date was very poorly understood by me, I had therefore decided to undertake journey through the much untrodden and equally unrevealed aspects of this problem. I humbly put before this profession my hectic days of the tour which I had undertaken to reach my destination. I have put the matter in much condensed form that would help those busy in this profession.

Farokh J. Master

DEDICATION

The book is humbly dedicated to my teacher
Dr. SARABHAI KAPADIA
B Sc., D.M.S. (Cal.)
Bombay

ENURESIS

Synonym : Bed-wetting

INTRODUCTION

The Ebers Papyrus documents that bed-wetting was well known in 1500 B.C. Enuresis is one of the most common and perplexing problems brought to the attention of the Homoeopath. By the 19th Century, doctors realised that. no matter what sort of treatment was suggested, if done with authority or zeal or kindliness, many cases of enuresis could be ameliorated. Today more is known about its causes and treatment possibilities, but enuresis still defies medical expertise. The ubiquity and frequency of this minor malady oblige it to be considered one of the most important pathologies of childhood. Further, in a considerable number of cases, enuresis persists into adulthood. A few cases have been seen in persons in late life who have never known dryness.

DEFINITION

Enuresis can be defined as bed-wetting or clothes-wetting in persons over the age of 3, who fail to inhibit the reflex to pass urine when the impulse is felt during waking hours and those who do not rouse from sleep of their own accord when the process is occurring during the sleeping state.

EPIDEMIOLOGY

Enuresis is found in all countries, among rich and poor in both sexes. It afflicts those in normal and sub-normal ranges of intelligence. No race is exempt. The study of enuretic population by Psychiatrists, Psychologists, Paediatricians and Homoeopaths suggest that boys are more likely than girls to suffer enuresis. The ratio is 2 : 1. The difference has been ascribed to social attitudes in child rearing, whereby girls are not permitted to be untidy, hence, they are trained to greater fastidiousness. Some argue that the incidence ratio reflects genetic considerations.

Researchers and clinicians agree, however, that those patients who are enuretic only at night are much less likely to have any associated or causative organic pathology. Since 80% of enuretics are only nocturnal in their habit, organicity must be sought more vigorously in one of every five cases; 15% of sufferers are diurnal enuretics only. It is in the last group that the physician must be hyperaware of the possibility of the organic cause.

Persons whose enuresis persists into adolescence show a greater frequency combinations with one or more of the following disturbances :

(1) Passive aggressive or Passive dependant reactions; (2) Past history of sleep walking ; (3) Family history of sleep walking ; (4) Inferior dentition as measured by decayed, filled or missing index ; (5) Chronic genito-urinary tract complaints (urgency, frequency, nocturia) and (6) Family history of enuresis.

However, in general, no known psychiatric diagnosis is associated with enuresis.

NORMAL DEVELOPMENT OF SPHINCTER CONTROL

The frequency of urination in babies varies from child to child. There is often a temporary phase of increased frequency at the age of about 21 months. At 2½ years there is often a retention span of about 5 hours. The retention span then rapidly increases with age.

Babies commonly empty the bowel and bladder immediately after a meal, especially in the first 8 months, and they can often be 'conditioned' to use the pottie any time after 2-3 months of age. This condition frequently breaks down as a result of teething or some disturbance of routine, particularly between 12 and 18 months. It is important to realize that there is no voluntary control at this time, for voluntary control does not begin till about 15-18 months of age.

The first indication of voluntary control is awareness at about 15 to 18 months of having passed urine, the child pointing it out to the mother. Shortly after the child is able to say 'No' with reasonable correctness when asked if he wants to urinate. He now begins to tell the mother just before he passes urine, but he does not give her time to 'catch' him. The urgency decreases as he grows older, and by 18-24 months he tells the mother in sufficient time for her to place him on the pottie. By 2-2½ years he is able to pull his pants down and go to the lavatory and may climb on to the lavatory seat unaided. Children at 2 to 2½ begin to take responsibility for not wetting their pants, and as a result the napkin is discarded during the day, but they are still wet by night. By 2½ the retention span is longer, and between 2½ and 3, if lifted out at 10 or 11 p.m. he is dry in the morning and the night time nappie is discarded. By 2½ two thirds are usually dry by day and half of them by night, by 3 years about 85% are dry at night, though occasional accidents may occur till he is 4 or older. He rarely soils his pants after age of two years, girls tend to acquire sphincter control earlier than boys.

MECHANISMS INVOLVED

The mechanisms relevant to the acquisition of sphincter control are mainly four—maturation, development, learning and conditioning :

(*i*) Maturation :

The mechanism of sphincter control is a complex one, and one must depend on the maturation of the nervous system. There is commonly a familar pattern ; just as some children are earlier or later than others in learning to sit, walk, talk or use their eyes or ears, so some children are earlier or later than others in controlling the bladder or bowel.

(*ii*) **Learning** :

Children learn to control the bladder partly by instruction and training. Training consists largely by helping the child when he is developmentally ready. As one famous poet said, "When the clock strikes certain hours, little pots are punctually applied to little botts".

(*iii*) **Conditioning** :

Here the babies empty the bladder when his buttocks feel the rim of the pottie.

AETIOLOGY AND BACKGROUND OF ENURESIS

The causes and background of enuresis are usually complex and often interrelated ; they include the following :

(*a*) *Delayed maturation.*

(*b*) *Faulty conditioning.* If the child is punished for not using the pottie when placed on it he will become conditioned against it and may refuse to use it.

(*c*) *Faulty learning.* If a mother fails to give her child an opportunity to empty the bladder when he first begins to announce that he wants to void, he is liable to be retarded in acquiring control.

(*d*) *The child's developing ego and personality.* From about 6 months onwards the child is developing his ego and his determination to be recognised as a person of importance. At 9 or 10 months he begins to repeat a performance laughed at. From about 12 months he characteristically enters the stage of negativism, so that if an attempt is made to try to force him to do anything against his will, in this case to use the pottie, he will refuse. Hence determined and over-enthusiastic efforts

The following investigations should be made :

(*i*) Blood pressure. Blood urea.

(*ii*) Biochemical and Microscopical examination of the urine.

(*iii*) Intravenous pyelogram.

(*vi*) Micturating cystogram.

CLINICAL FEATURES

The observation of cloth-wetting or bed-wetting is made very easily. However, the observer cannot tell whether there is an organic cause, or whether the person is enuretic. Usually, the person who brings the chief complaint can offer testimony as to the wetting episodes and their pattern of occurrence. In the majority of cases there is no difficulty in deciding that the wetting is a case of enuresis.

There are two general categories of enuretics—the primary, also called the persistant enuretic and the secondary, also called transient or neurotic enuretic. Four-fifths of all enuretics are primary, which means that a period of sustained dryness has never developed and that the patient has never known the confident feeling of retiring without the worry of enuresis. The secondary enuresis appears after a person has stopped wetting. A neurotic conflict, such as a birth of a sibling, or a transient emotional stress, such as making an adjustment to military service may precipitate enuresis. The physician must note whether the enuretic episodes are diurnal, nocturnal, or both diurnal and nocturnal. It has been estimated that at least 1 of every 1,000 enuretics has an associated encopresis, the involuntary passage of faeces.

Adult enuretics are able to describe heart-rending inconveniences and situations occasioned by the persistence of their habit. They have had such limitations as not having been able to go away to school and being able to stay overnight with a loved one. Nevertheless many adult enuretics are married and lead usual existences.

In enuretic boys there is often a mother-son relationship in which the child continues his enuresis because of the unconscious expectations and wishes of the mother. The mother often has depreciatory attitudes towards that make her demand that her son be both ineffective and rebellious.

Female enuretics, on the other hand, have a strong attachment to their fathers. Just as the male enuretic may be a mother's boy, the female enuretic may be a father's girl.

COURSE AND PROGNOSIS

Medically, enuresis can be considered a benign disorder that has a strong tendency to self correction. Hence, the time honoured counsel to parents that the enuresis will cease when the child grows up seems, with certain exceptions, to be true.

Although most children are dry by age 10, any child who is enuretic should be treated early, since, at present, it is impossible to distinguish the child who will continue to suffer enuresis into adolescence and adulthood.

DIAGNOSIS

Although the cause and management of enuresis baffle physicians, the diagnosis is relatively easy. The patient can tell the physician about involuntary urine passage.

A homoeopath who sees an enuretic child must be sure that the patient has had a thorough physical examination and urinalysis. He must also take a complete medical history and then discover the characteristics of the wetting pattern.

TREATMENT

No treatment method is so successful as to win universal endorsement. The clinician is faced with a disorder whose cause is not understood and whose differential diagnosis is deceptively complex. The management of a case of enuresis is difficult. The following are the array of approaches available with homoeopath. The selection of appropriate method depends on the individual circumstances. Usually a homoeopath selects a combination of methods.

I. PLACEBOS

In homoeopathic literature marvellous cases of success are reported by using placebos.

Case: A boy aged 12 yrs. History of enuresis since 10 years. The boy was the only child and was very nervous and sickly. He had been given a lot of homoeopathic and allopathic treatment in the past without any benefit. He was warned by me that if he does not stop wetting the bed then the surgeon will operate on him. Also the cut of the surgery will be from head to foot. He was also given a bottle of S.L. pills and told that if he desires to prevent this major surgery then he should take 2 pills, three times a day for a fortnight He took the treatment for three months from me but till today he has spoiled the bed only twice. H is still under observation. The success of placebo therapy largely depends on the raport between the homoeopath and the patient. The only demerit of this therapy is when the patient discovers the hoax.

II. CONDITIONING DEVICES

The most effective way of banishing the symptom of bed-wetting is to use a conditioning device that awakens the patient by an alarm bell or a buzzer as soon as a drop of urine contacts a wire pad on which he is sleeping. The conditioning process quickly leads to the cessation of bed-wetting, since the patient learns to awaken and void before the stimulates of the bell or buzzer.

Disadvantages : After years of experience I have come to the conclusion that conditioning devices are of little help and relapse is bound to occur.

The treatment according to many homoeopaths is cruel, punitive and insensitive. The other practical problem is that when the buzzer sounds it also awakens other children sleeping in the same room thereby spoiling the peaceful sleep.

Also false alarms are very common because few children perspire a lot and these very drops of perspiration stimulate the alarm.

PSYCHOTHERAPY

Critical to the management of any case of enuresis is psychotherapy. The psychiatrist must be supportive and must be capable of promoting and sustaining feelings of confidence and hope in the patient.

On guard, the psychotherapy involves encouragement and patience both in the consultation room and at home. The parents must be partners in the process so that, with their co-operation the patient feels that there are attitudinal changes in regard to bed-wetting.

DRUGS

The array of drugs includes anticholinergics, sympathomimetics, sedatives, relaxants, diuretics, anti-diuretics and anti-depressants.

At the present time, anti-depressants are the drugs of choice in the treatment of enuresis for the allopathic physicians. However, I have seen in my practice that those patients who were given tricyclic anti-depressants, including amitriptyline and nortriptyline by their family physician, the children developed many side-effects like dysuria, retention, dryness of mouth, dizziness, headache, constipation, loss of appetite, weight loss, sleep disturbance and above all *drug addiction*.

I am sure after going through the long list of side-effects no homoeopath with reasonable mind will ever think of using modern drugs for his patient.

BLADDER TRAINING

For a long time it has been known that some enuretics have smaller than normal functional bladder capacities. That fact led urologists to promote the treatment method of bladder training. In this therapy the patient is asked to quantify his ability to drink measured volumes of fluid and to withhold the urination for as long as possible. The desired result is that the patient becomes able to withold increasingly larger volumes of fluid over longer periods of time. Hence, the vesicle is trained and becomes adaptive in accommodating greater quantities of urine. At night the patient's heightened threshold for retention eliminates the problem of bed-wetting.

SLEEP INTERRUPTION

In view of the hypersomnia observed in enuretics long before the era of laboratory sleep research. it has been suggested that parents wake up the child to void during the night. Favourable responses may have been due to the focussed concern by the parents and the child, as well as to postive behaviourial reinforcement.

HYPNOSIS

Hypnosis has been used in the treatment of enuretics in Europe and in the United States. Like all treatment methods in enuresis, there are enthusiastic claims and counter claims concerning its success.

REPERTORY OF ENURESIS

1. Urination ; Involuntary ; night (Incontinence in bed) :

Acon^2	Aethusa^1	Am-c^2	Anac^1
Anan^1	Apis^3	Apocy^2	Arg-m^2
Arg-n^3	Arn^3	Ars^3	Aur^2
Aur-m^1	Aur-s^1	Bar-c^2	Bar-m^1
Bella^3	Benz-acid^3	Bry^2	Cact^1
Calc^3	Canth^1	Carh-s^2	Carb-v^3
Caust^3	Cham^3	Chen-v^1	Chin^2
Chlo^2	Cimex^1	Cina^3	Coca^2
Con^2	Crot-c^1	Cub^2	Cupr^1
Dulc^2	Equis^3	Eup-pur^2	Ferr^3
Ferr-ars^1	Ferr-i^1	Ferr-phos^2	Fl-acid^2
Gels^1	Graph^3	Iep^3	Hyos^2
Ign^2	K-br^1	K-c^2	K-p^3
Kreos^3	Lac-c^2	Lac-d^1	Lyc^2
Mag-c^1	Mag-m^2	Mag-p^2	Mag-s^1
Med^2	Merc^3	Mur-ac^1	Nat-ars^2
Nat-c^2	Nat-m^3	Nat-phos^1	Nit-acid^2
Nux-vomica^2	Op^3	Ox-acid^1	Petro^2
Phos-ac^2	Phos^2	Physal^1	Plan^3
Podo^2	Psar^2	Puls^3	Qyass^1
Rhus-ar^1	Rhus-t^3	Ruta^2	Sabal^2
Sanic^2	Santon^1	Sars^2	Sec^1
Seneg^2	Sep^3	Sil^3	Spig^2
Squil^1	Staph^2	Stram^2	Sul^3
Syph^1	Tab^1	Ter^1	Thuja^2
Thuya^2	Thyr^2	Tab^3	Uran^2
Veret^1	Verb^2	Viol-t^2	Zn^1

2. Morning towards, agg :
   Am-c[1] Cact[1] Chlo[1] Zinc[1]
3. Morning, agg : Carbo-veg[1]
4. At night. Worse in Autumn :
   Puls[2]
5. At night in boys of light complexion :
   Sep[2]
6. At night. in fat children, red face, sweat easily and catch cold : Calc[2].
7. At night children in later part of night, even if they have urinated during night and drank no water :
   Chloral[1]
8. At night in nervous children :
   Gels[2]
9. At night in children of Phosphorus build :
   Phos[2]
10. At night pale, lean children with large abdomen, who love sugar and highly seasoned food and abhar to be washed :
    Sul[1]
11. At night in scrofulous and syphillitic children :
    Kal-iod[1]
12. At night floods bed five or six times :
    Ferrum[1]
13. At night after great fright two years age :
    Phos[1]
14. At night particularly in little girl :
    Puls[1]
15. At night from infancy in girl at 16 :
    Nux-vom[1]
16. At night after blow, upon head :
    Sil[1]

17. At night during fullmoon, obstinate case :
Psorinum^{2}

18. At night from nervous irritation :
Magn-p^{3}

19. At night old man after dropsy :
Aur-mur^{2}

20. At night in onanists :
Sep^{2}

21. At night while at rest :
Rhus^{2}

22. At night especially during first sleep :
Caust^{2} Cina^{2} Phos-ac^{2} Sep^{3}

23. At night 1st sleep fairly flood the bed :
Phos-ac^{2}

24. At night during 1st sleep from which child is roused with difficulty :
Kreos^{2}

25. At night spasmodic form :
Arg-met^{2}

26. At night weakness of sphincter :
Ferrum-ph^{1}, Gels^{2}, Plant^{2}

27. At night from worms :
Uran-n^{2}

28. At night with ascarides :
Ferr^{2}

29. At night in children with worms and in chorea :
Sil^{2}

30. At night for two years :
Sul^{1}

31. Midnight to morning :
Plan^{1}

32. After 5 A.M. :
Cact^{1}

33. Adult of :

Kali-carb[1]

34. Bed is wet almost as soon as child goes to sleep, always during 1st sleep :

Sepia[1]

35. Bladder paralysis in children with affection of head :

Hyos[2]

Causes incontinence : Kali-Phos[2]

36. Cathetarization from :

Mag-phos[1]

37. In children with acidity of stomach :

Nat-phos[1]

38. In children who grow too rapidly :

Phos[2]

39. In children where urine is scanty, acrid and loaded with uric acids and its deposits :

Plat[2]

40. In weakly children :

China[2]

41. Cause without any except habit :

Equis

42. Difficult to waken the child :

Bella[2] Kreos[2]

43. Digestive disturbance :

Benz-ac[1] Nux-vomica[2]
Puls[1]

44. Dreaming of urination :

Kreos[2], Lac-c[1], Lyc[1], Merc-i-f[1]
Seneg[2] Sep[2] Sulph[1]

45. Dribling in boy :

Rhux-tox[2]

46. Dribling nocturnal and diurnal enuresis :

Nux-vomica[1]

47. During 1st sleep, child aroused with difficulty :

Caust Kreosot Sep[2]

48. During fullmoon, intractable causes eczematous history :

Psori

49. Enuresis (see wetting bed) :

Can-sat[1], Kali-p[1], Nit-ac[1], Puls[1]

Rhus-t[1] (Bary-c, Bry, Spong)

50. Enuresis, in old age :

Sec[1]

51. Enuresis at night with profuse sweat :

Bell[1]

52. Enuresis head throw back during sleep :

Hep-s[1]

53. Enuresis invol. micturition at night in bed :

Petrol[1]

54. Enuresis frequent micturition at night (during pregnancy) :

Podophy[1]

55. Enuresis wetting of bed :

Hep-s

56. Enuresis of children :

Benz-acid, Kali-p

57. Enuresis at night in scrofulus or syphil children :

Kali-iod

58. Enuresis with thirst :

Acon[1]

59. Enuresis alternate with dysuria :

Gels[1]

60. Enuresis nocturnal :

Graph, Verbascum

61. Feeling of weakness in bladder and genitals with fear of wetting bed :

Alumina[1]

62. First sleep :

Bez-ac[1], Caust[3], Cina[2], Kreosot[2]
Phos-ac[2], Sep[3]

63. From fright two years ago :
Phos

64. Habit the only ascertainable cause :
Equis[1]

65. Head blow on from :
Silicea[1]

66. H/o Sycosis :
Med[1]

67. Hysterical :
Ign[1], Val-m[1]

68. Invol. discharge of urine at night wetting bed :
Am-c[1], Carbo-veg[1], Caust[1], Cina[1], Puls[1]
Senega[1], Sepia[1], Silcea[1], Sulph[1]

69. Invol. micturition at night in bed (especially in little girls) while coughing or passing flatus :
Puls[1]

70. Measles after : Puls[2]

71. Moon full :
Cina[1], Psor[1]

72. Old man :

Apoc[1], Benz-ac[1], Kali-p[2]
Sec[1]

73. Paretic condition of sphincter muscle of bladder causing enuresis and spasmodic retention of urine :
Gels[1]

74. Pregnancy in :
Podo[1]

75. Sleep during first :
Benz-ac[2], Caust[2], Kreosot[2]
Phos-aci, Sep[3]

76. Sleep during last part :
Chlo-h

77. Spasmodic enuresis :
Arg-m^{3}, Bella^{1}, Canth^{1}, Caps^{1}, Caust^{1}, Cina^{1}
Coloc^{1}, Gels^{2}, Hyos^{1}, Ign^{1}, Lach^{1}, Lyco^{1}
Nux-v^{2}, Op^{1}, Puls^{1}, Rhus-t^{1}, Verel^{1}

78. Tangible cause except habit when there is not :
Equis^{3}

79. Waking difficulties :
Bella^{1}, Chlo-hyd^{1}, Kreos^{2}

80. Weakness of sphincter of bladder especially in children urine passes involuntarily, especially during first sleep at night, also invol. from slightest excitment during day :
Causticum^{1}

81. Weak children in :
Cina^{2}

82. Weak or paretic sphincter vesica :
Apoc^{1}, Bell^{2}, Caust^{2}, Con^{1}, Ferr-p^{1}
Gels^{2}, Nux-v^{1}, Rars^{1}, Sabal^{1}, Sec^{1}, Strych^{2}

83. Wet-bed, restless, starts in sleep :
Bella

84. Wets bed at night, wakes up with urging but cannot retain urine :
Kreosotum^{1}

85. Wetting bed at night
Apoc^{1}

86. Wetting bed at night in children :
Equis^{1}, Kali-phos^{1}, Petroleum^{1}

87. Wetting bed at night children from worms :
Cina^{1}

88. Worms :
Cina^{1}, Santon^{2}, Sul^{1}

Drug	*Time of Enuresis*	*Sleep Pattern*	*Cause*	*Character of Urine*	*Constitution*	*Tempera-ment*	*Accompani-ment*
(*1*)	(*2*)	(*3*)	(*4*)	(*5*)	(*6*)	(*7*)	(*8*)
Bella-dona	Generally after mid-night or to-wards early morning. Daytime	Half opened eyes. Restless sleep with sudden starts ; moaning and screaming during sleep. Grinding, ster-torous sleep. Somnolence, sle-epy yet cannot slecp. Sleeps with hands under the head.	Eating too much sugar. Paralysis of bladder.	Yellow and scanty. Tur-bid. Dark red. Profu-sed deposits of phos-phate. Stron-gly acidic.	Scrofulous	Anxiety[2]. Quarrelsome. Bilious. Lymphatic.	Easy pers-piration, faeces escape while urina-ting, sensa-tion of worms in the bladder.
Benzoic Acid	During mid-night in girls.	Starts up. Awakes with breathless-		High colou-red. Smells	Gouty & Rheumatic	Confused ideas cross.	Sheets are unusually

(1)	(2)	(3)	(4)	(5)	(6)	(7)	(8)
(Where Nitrum fails.)		ness and palpitation.		like that of horse's. Sour. Ammoniacal. Hot. Profuse. Alkaline.	Diathesis		brown stained.
Cal. Carb	Enuresis in bed; when walking After midnight. Hysterical and spasm of the bladder.	Screams and cannot be pacified. Nightmares. Fearful & fantastic dreams. Snoring.	Masturbation. Loss of fluids. Fright. Egotism.	Dark brown. Strong odour. White sediment. Offensive.	Fat, Flabby children with red faces. Tendency to catch cold. Leucophlegmatic. Scrofulous. Plethoric. Gouty. Delicate.	Dull. Delayed, confused fearful, forgetful. Leucophlegmatic. Nervous bilious Sanguine.	Easy Parpiratic Pica. Pitutary and thyroid dysfunctions. Tendency to take cold.

(1)	(2)	(3)	(4)	(5)	(6)	(7)	(8)
Causti-cum	During first sleep. During cold weather. During cold nights.	Restless sleep. Starts laughs and cries. Drowsy—can hardly keep awake. Sensitive wakes up. No sensation of passing urine; scarcely believes untill he makes sure of sense of touch.	Fright, Grief, Nightwatch-ing. Retention.	Deposits of Urates. Cloudy Uric acid bloody.	Children with black hair & eyes & rigid fibres. Delicate skin. Hydrogenoid scrofulous.	Nervous girls. Slow in learning.	Warts weak-ness, stools passed in standing position.
Cina	During second half of the sleep. Full moon.	Restless during sleep. Lies on abdomen, knee-chest. Talks, cries, screames,	Worms.	Copious. Turns milky on standing. Turbid white.	Big, fat, rosy and scrofulous.	Restless. Touchy. Capricious.	Hungry, worms, Grinds teeth. Convulsions.

(1)	(2)	(3)	(4)	(5)	(6)	(7)	(8)
		wakes frightened. Hangs his head to one side. Will not sleep unless rocked.					
Equisetum hyemale.	Day and night.	Dreams of seeing crowds of people.	Habitual. (no cause known)	Clear, light colour. Profuse. Scanty.	Habitual Enuretics.		Dyspepsia.
Ferrmet	More frequently in day time than at night 5/6 night standing.	Sleepy : of debility. Restless lies on back. Vivid unpleasant, fell into water.	Weakness of the sphincter, vesieac. Worms.	Light colour of stains the sheets very dark and smell strong ammonia. Hot profuse. Mucous sediment.	False plethora pale. Emaciated. Weak, delicate, Lymphatic. Haemorrhagic diathesis.	Sensitive. Excitable. Sanguine. Choleric, Phlegmatic.	Allergies changeable.

(1)	(2)	(3)	(4)	(5)	(6)	(7)	(8)
Kali-brom	2 a.m. New moon.	Somnambulism. Starts. Deep sleep, Moans, Cries, Grinding. Horrible dreams.	Nightmare Worries. Spasmodic.	Pale, Profuse, Sugar^x	Obese	Depressed, Forgetful, weepy. Lymphatic. Sanguine.	Thirst, Appetite, Constipation, Tender liver, Diabetic Headache[3].
Kali-phos		Night terrors. Somnambulism. Amorous dreams. Restlessness. Wakes up with fright.	Nervous debility.	Saffron yellow, milky.		Nervous, sensitive, depressed, gloomy, forgetful, fearful.	Diabetics
Kreo-sotom	First part of night.	Dreams of falling poisoned, fire, of urination in a descent manner. Wakes with uri-		Copious. Pale urine. Offensive. Brown, red sediment.	Overgrown poorly developed children. Marasmus.	Capricious Leucophlegmatic.	Black caries.

(1)	(2)	(3)	(4)	(5)	(6)	(7)	(8)
		nating from deep sleep but cannot retain. Restless, Tosses. Would not sleep until caressed & fondled.			Lean, thin, blonde, brunettes.		
Lac-Caninum	Screams+ Lies with one leg flexed and other stretched.	She dreams of urinating.		Scanty, dark. thick, reddish sediment.	Dark hair, eyes, Rheumatic enlarged glands.	Forgetful, cross, irritable.	Diphtheria. sore throat.
Mercurius	Night 3 am.	Sleepless of anxiety. Restlessness, dreams of water, thieves, animals.	Paralysis	Copious/ scanty urinates more than he drinks. mixed with	Tendency to sweat profusely. Light hair with lax skin and	Nervous. Lack of will. Lymphatic. Choleric.	Easily suppurative tonsilbitis, Thirst.++ Sweat.++

(1)	(2)	(3)	(4)	(5)	(6)	(7)	(8)
				blood white sediment. Strong smelling. Staining diaper. Hot acrid.	muscles. Scrofulous strong, florid complexion. Lively brunette.	Melancholic, Sanguine.	Tongue indented Stomatitis.
Arg-met.	Nocturnal (Spasmodic forms)	Restless sleep, anxious frightful dreams, Screams.	Diabetics	Turbid. Pale. Fetid, profuse, sweat odour.	Lean, thin, robust, anaemic. Rheumatic.	Anticipatory, Anxiety, Fear, depressed, irritable.	
Bar-c.	Night	Talks in sleep. Twitchings. Lies on one side.		Scanty, dark brown. Copious.	Dwarfish, Retàrded, Scrofulous.	Absent-minded.	Oversensitive to all. Impression. Tendency to take cold.

(1)	*(2)*	*(3)*	*(4)*	*(5)*	*(6)*	*(7)*	*(8)*
Nat-mur	Alternate days. Full moon.	Somnambulism. Starts and talks in sleep. Dreams of robbers, vivid, frightful, tosses.	Fright, Grief.	Clear, watery red sediment, turbid, dark.	Lean, thin, scrofulous, brown hair, blue eyes. Dark complexion.	Awkward, Irritable, Delayed mental and physical nervous, sanguine.	Hopeless. school girl's headache, Waterbrash, Diabetics.
Phosphorus		Somnambulism. Dreams of fire, lewd, vivid, business. She couldn't finish. Starts in sleep. Lies on right side.	Anger, Grief. Diabetes, During Typhoid.	Profuse, Pale, Haematuria, Albumin, Watery, Turbid, brick-dust sediment offensive.	Lean, thin, tall, beautiful. Grow too rapidly, Gouty, Scrofulous, Fair, delicate eyelashes and smooth hair, Haemorrhagic.	Sensitive, Nervous, Sanguine. Quick, lively perceptions.	Craving cold things. Wants to be magnetised.

(1)	(2)	(3)	(4)	(5)	(6)	(7)	(8)
Pulsatilla	in little girls in Autumn.	Lies with hands over head or crossed on abdomen and feet drawn up. Talks, screams. Restless. Tosses. Dreams-confused, frightful.	Anger. Spasm. Measles after.	Mucus, scanty, red brown, profuse.	Fair complexion. Sandy hair, blue eyes. Pale face. Scrofulous, robust.	Mild, timid, weepy. Indecisive, slow, phlegmatic, sanguine, Hysterical.	Thirstlessness.
Rhus-tox	Night-Midnight in boys.	Dreams of exertion, fire; blood. Restless, tossing.		Dark, Turbid, Scanty, Hot.	In boys, Rheumatic Scrofulous, brown, complexion, lean, small stature, tall, slender.	Anxious Restless, confused, Hypochondrical Sanguine.	

(1)	*(2)*	*(3)*	*(4)*	*(5)*	*(6)*	*(7)*	*(8)*
Sepia	First sleep	Talks loud, Wakes up. Restless. Dreams of urinating anxious.	Anger, Vexation,	Foul, Sour, White, milky Red scanty, cloudy.	Delicate, Plethoric, Yellow complexion, leucophlegmatic, in boys of ligh complexion with onanist. Dark-hair, rigid fibres, Scrofulous.	Nervous, Irritable, Sanguine, Bilious, Jovial.	
Silicea	Moon phases	Somnambulism. Talks loudly, laughs. Dreams of Lascivious, pleasant, murders, Restless, Wakes up frightened.	Worms, Blow upon head. Diabetes.	Purulent, Bloody, profuse.	Emaciated, large head, open fontanells, scrofulous, Rachitis.	Sensitive, want of grit, Lymphatic, Torpid, Phlegmatic, Sanguine.	Night sweats, Constipation.

(1)	*(2)*	*(3)*	*(4)*	*(5)*	*(6)*	*(7)*	*(8)*
Sul-phur		Sleeps in catnaps, talks, jerks and twiches in sleep. Wakes up singing. vivid dreams.		Greasy particles.	Scrofulous untidy		
Thuja		Dreams of death of falling from a height.			Hydrogenoid, Lymphoid.	Nervous, Hurried, fixed ideas, irritable.	
Tub-bov		Dreams of vivid, frightful, restless, tosses, screams. Awakes in horror.		Sediments	Light complexion, narrow chested. Scrofulous.	Sensitive.	
Zinc		Screams, jerks, starts, Somnambulism.					

BIBLIOGRAPHY

1. The Normal Child—by Ronald S. Illingworth. VI Ed. 1975, Chapt. 23, p. 230.

. Abnormal Psychology and Modern Life—James C. Coleman. VVV Ed. 1981, Chap. 15, p. 548.

3. Essential Paediatrics—D. P. Ghai, 1981 Ed. Chapt. 2, p. 23.

4. Handbook of Paediatrics—Henry Silver—Henry Kemps, Henry Brui, XIII Edi., p. 171.

5. A Short Textbook of Paediatrics—Suraj Gupta, III Edi. 1982, p. 284.

6. Children's Diseases by John R. Short, O.P. Grey, J.A. Dodge, V. Edi. 1978, Chap. 117, p. 476.

7. Practical Paediatric Problems—James H. Hutchison, V. Edi. 1980, Chap. 27, p. 622.

8. Diseases of Children—Hugh Jolley, IV Edi. 1981, Chap. 18, p. 413.

9. Current Paediatric, Henry Kampe, Silver, Donough Obrein, VI Edi. Chap. 23, p. 674.

10. Comprehensive Textbook of Psychiatry, Vol. I, II and III-Caplan, Friedman, Sodlock, III Edi.

11. Textbook of Paediatrics—Nelson—XI Edi. p-89.

12. Hab. Glem. Vol. XLV, No. 2, Feb. 1978.

13. Maxwell, MD, Seldrup J : Imipremina in the treatment of Childhood Euresis. Practitioner, 207 : 809, 1971.

14. Oppel, WC, Harper, PA, Rider, RV : Social, Psychological and neurological factors associated with nocturnal enuresis. Paediatrics, 42 : 627, 1968.

15. Silberstein, RM, Blackmon, S : Differential Diagnosis and treatment of enuresis. American Journal of Psychiatry, 121 : 1204. 1965.

16. Stanfield, B: Enueresis : Its pathogenesis and management. Clinical Paediatrics (Phila) 11 : 343, 1972.

17. Werry, JS, Cohrssen, J : Enuresis : An etiologic and therapeutic study. Journal of Pediatrics, 67 : 423, 1965.

